HOW TO GET OVER THE STIGMA OF MENTAL ILLNESS

LEARN WHAT CHALLENGES YOU WILL FACE

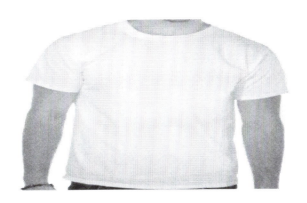

PATRICIA A CARLISLE

Introduction

I want to thank you and congratulate you for choosing the book, *"HOW TO GET OVER THE STIGMA OF MENTAL ILLNESS: LEARN WHAT CHALLENGES YOU WILL FACE "*.

Mental illness is a psychological pattern that occurs in an individual and it causes distress and disability. This medical condition disturbs a person's thinking, daily doings, feeling and ability to maintain with others. Serious mental illnesses include major depression, schizophrenia, bipolar disorder, obsessive-compulsive disorder (OCD), panic disorder, posttraumatic stress disorder (PTSD), and borderline personality disorder. The most important thing is that it can be recovered.

Medical illnesses can take many forms, just as physical illnesses do. Mental illnesses are still feared and misunderstood by many people, but the fear will disappear as people learn more about them. But in order to be fearless you must get the following information.

Mental illness is very common. One out of every four people in Britain is dealing with a mental illness. Mental illnesses are some of the least understood conditions in society. As a result of this condition, many people face prejudice and discrimination in their everyday lives. However, most people can lead productive and fulfilling lives with appropriate treatment and support.

For some people, drugs and other medical treatments are helpful, but for others they are not. Medical treatment may only be a part of what helps recovery, and not necessarily the main part. It is not a fault of someone rather this is not a sign of weakness, and it's not something to be ashamed of.

Persons suffering from any of the severe mental disorders present with a variety of symptoms that may include inappropriate anxiety, disturbances of thought and perception, deregulation of mood, and cognitive dysfunction. Most of these symptoms may be relatively specific to a particular diagnosis or cultural influence.

For example, disturbances of thought and perception are most commonly associated with schizophrenia. Similarly, severe disturbances in expression of affect and regulation of mood are most commonly seen in depression and in bipolar disorder. However, it is not uncommon to see psychotic symptoms in patients diagnosed with mood disorders, or to see mood-related symptoms in patients diagnosed with schizophrenia. Symptoms associated with mood, anxiety, thought process, or cognition may occur in any patient at some point during his or her illness.

So what is stigma. "Stigma" describes the shame, fear and discrimination that result from stereotypes surrounding mental illness. It can affect people with a mental illness psychologically and even economically, when it comes to finding housing and employment. Stigma can cause family tension and rejection. It also leads to fear, mistrust and violence against people with mental illness.

Thank you again for choosing this book, I hope you enjoy it!

ABOUT THE AUTHOR

Patricia A. Carlisle, MSW, CBT

Patricia Carlisle- a Master in Social Work and Cognitive Behavioral Therapist (CBT) gives out an expression of how important it is for an individual to take into consideration the concept of self-assessment to know what human, technical and conceptual skills they posses to perform or to achieve what they desire, or to deal with everyday life. However, every particular group of people has their own unique set of ideas, traditions and events including the frame of mind according to which people perform but there are many who faces problems and fail to maintain a healthy mind set affecting their behaviors and performance to those around them.

People like Patricia Carlisle are among those who have felt this urge of serving people and helping them out of their mental crisis towards a healthy life. She has experienced some close encounters in her personal life regarding mental health issues in her family and friends that has encouraged her to pursue this as her career.

Currently Patricia Carlisle is serving as a Certified On-Line Cognitive Behavioral Therapist with an extensive 15years of experience using Cognitive-Behavior Therapy Techniques. She envisions a world where everyone gets mental health treatment with no mental health stigma and to make it real she has already set up her own Holistic Measure Online Comprehensive Behavioral Healthcare Company after retiring from The Nord

Center in The Partial Hospitalization Program (PHP) Dept for 5 years and Murtis H. Taylor Mental Health Center as a mental health counselor, psychological support technician and case manager for 10 years to emulsify her skills more professionally.

Along with this, she has wrote down her passion as a clinician in 25 or more short books to help individuals and families get their life back, freeing them of the restraints of negative thinking, anxiety and depression by using different approaches. She is highly appreciated among her clients for her flexibility and professionalism of dealing with them graciously. To reach her, make use of her direct website address: http://therapist2013.wix.com/e-therapy . As she is ready to inspire hope and contribute to health and well-being by providing the best online health care through comprehensive practice, education and research.

TABLE OF CONTENT

Chapter 1

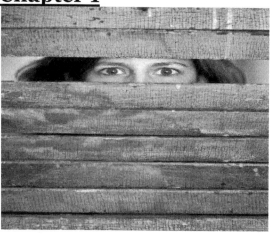

THE IMPACT OF STIGMA

It is no secret that mental illness is surrounded by stigma. There are numerous negative terms used to describe people with mental illnesses; many of these terms are used in everyday conversation. We are so familiar with them in fact, most people have no idea that they are furthering the stigma by using them.

Think about some of these common terms: crazy, nuts, wacko, psycho. These terms are use to describe people, ideas, events, etc. But also to label those with legitimate medical conditions. By referring to people in this way it casually toss them into a group without really trying to understand them, or their illness.

The fact is, 1 in 4 American adults can be diagnosed with a mental illness in any given year. That's 25% of the adult U.S. population. Chances are you know someone who has a mental illness. Studies have shown that those with mental illnesses can recover faster, and better with the support of family and friends. Yet, many people choose to hide their disorders from their closest family members, co-workers, and social circles. Why? Because of stigma.

Stigma makes these individuals feel ashamed of their disorder, fearful of how people's perceptions of them may change. They even fear knowing themselves; which is why it often takes people so long to seek treatment for a mental disorder. When terms like "crazy," "nuts," "wacko," etc. are so predominant, you can see why someone with a diagnosis would be fearful of revealing it.

In this way, stigma hurts an individual already dealing with the pain of a mental illness. But the impact is far greater than just the individual. If stigma prevents someone from seeking help for a mental illness, their illness may become worse. This can affect their family life, job, or school performance, and social network. Left untreated, a person may lose their job, family and friends. An astounding number of homeless individuals suffer with mental illness. There are high levels of mentally ill individuals in jails as well (on mostly non-violent charges).

In our society, stigma has an enormous impact. At best, it can cause someone to have to suffer silently with their mental health problem. At its worse, it can cause job loss, family disruption, homelessness, and incarceration. Both extremes are unacceptable.

There are many things we can all do to eliminate stigma and create a healthier community. First is to become educated about mental health, and the disorders that affect so many people. Stigma often arises from misconceptions and fears. Second, is to eliminate negative slang terms. Use "people first" language i.e. "a person with schizophrenia," instead of just "crazy." By learning about mental illness and being respectful of those with these common medical conditions, we can make huge progress towards eliminating stigma.

W hat Are The Causes Of Mental Illness

The exact cause of most mental illnesses is unknown, but there are many known factors at play. These can be biological, psychological or environmental. The cause varies from person to person, and it can be complicated. For most people who suffer from mental illnesses, the cause is some combination of these factors.

Genetic Factors

Most mental illnesses run in families. Studies have shown that there is a definite genetic factor. While your family history doesn't necessarily cause you to have the illness as well, it does put you at greater risk for developing it. In the case of schizophrenia, for example, people with close relatives that have this disorder are ten times more likely to develop it themselves. Chronic depression and bipolar disorder are similar.

Chemical Imbalance

Neurotransmitters are chemicals in the brain through which the brain communicates with the nerves. When these chemicals are not working properly, the brain doesn't function regularly, and this abnormal functioning leads to mental illness. This is why medications are used to treat symptoms. They restore normal brain functioning.

Early Development

Neglect or abuse in early life can lead to serious mental problems in adulthood. Severe emotional, physical and sexual abuse can all be contributing factors. The loss of a parent or any other traumatic event can lead to lifelong mental problems.

Long-Term Drug Use

There's a strong connection between drug use and mental illness. It's often hard to tell if the person is self-medicating to get rid of the symptoms or the drug triggers the symptoms. Marijuana, cocaine, amphetamines, psychedelic drugs such as LSD, alcohol and even seemingly harmless caffeine have all been linked to mental disorders. Long-term abuse of any substance can lead to anxiety, depression and paranoia.

Disease or Injury

Traumatic brain injury or exposure to toxins in the womb can cause mental illnesses. Lead in paint has been found to cause mental problems and certain foods are shown to contribute to ADHD. Infections that affect the brain can cause damage to areas involved in personality and thinking. The effect of disease and injury on the brain is not well understood because researchers have few chances to study real-life cases.

Life Experiences

Any kind of trauma that is either extremely stressful or persistent can lead to mental problems. The death of someone close to you, the experience of war, long-term harassment, working too hard or even being unemployed for too long can cause mental problems.

Society and Culture

Societal factors also contribute. There is a higher level of mental illness among immigrants, the poor, and people who lack social cohesion. Many blame the hectic pace of modern life, and the dissolution of traditional values for the rise in psychological disorders. Racial oppression can also be a factor. However, there is little scientific evidence to support these social and cultural factors.

Chapter 2

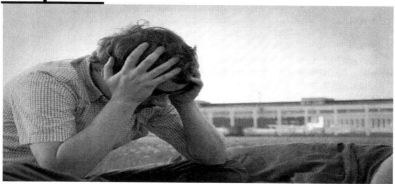

MENTAL ILLNESS CHALLENGES AND STIGMA

Mental illness is an enigma. It is everywhere all the time and we don't recognize it. When it gets to a point where it affects the life of the individual, and hence the family and friends, someone starts to notice. But it often takes a long time for all involved to really notice. We human beings have a tendency to deny things that we do not like, or are afraid to deal with, and so we use many techni☐ues to justify it.

For the most part mental illness is hard to recognize and hard to diagnose. In description mental illness is the sum of the devices that we use to avoid facing the truth about what is happening in our lives. Therefore the people closest to the ill person end up helping them to use those devices, and usually suffer themselves from emotional stress. It's a ripple affect.

And just for the record, all addictions are a form of mental illness. There is a stigma attached to mental illness. Sometimes for years people will all work together to keep it ☐uiet, or to pretend that it is just a personality trait. It becomes like an elephant in the middle of the room that everyone walks around as if it did not exist.

First of all, why is there a stigma attached to it? We all have permission to get cancer or heart disease without the world rejecting us. But get a mental disorder and people scatter like ants so that they won't be associated with someone 'crazy'. We are the crazy ones because we can help, and we don't.

HOW TO GET OVER THE STIGMA OF MENTAL ILLNESS

Stigma refers to the condition in which someone judges you depending on any particular personal trait. The sad part is that most of the people who suffer from mental illness face such a stigma □uite often. Stigma of mental illness can be both direct and obvious, for instance, when someone comments negatively on your mental condition or treatment; or subtle, such as a person assuming that you might be violent or unstable due to an underlying health condition. Some patients may even judge themselves. The most common detrimental effects of stigma include:

- Lack of understanding by family, friends, co-workers, or others.
- Reluctance to seek help or treatment.
- Discrimination at school, or work or in the society.
- Problems in finding housing opportunities.
- Fewer opportunities for work, school, or social activities, or trouble finding housing.
- Harassment, bullying, or physical violence.
- Health insurance which doesn't offer coverage for mental illnesses.
- Having a belief that you will never succeed in any challenge, and that you are incapable of improving your condition.

Here are 13 ways you can help a person with mental illness cope with the stigma related to their condition.

1. **Get The Right Treatment For Them:** Most mental patients are reluctant to admit they suffer from any kind of medical condition for which they need treatment. Help them to overcome their fear of being 'labeled' as a mental patient, which often prevent them from getting help. Treatment of the condition can be extremely helpful as it can help in identifying the root of the problem, and in reducing symptoms which often hinder one's personal life or work.

2. **Don't Allow The Stigma To Develop Shame And Self-Doubt In The Mental Patient:** It is not necessary that stigma will always come from someone else. Some people believe that their connection is being caused due to their own personal weakness. Taking the help of a psychologist, encouraging interaction with others, and educating them about their mental condition will help them to overcome self-judgment and gain self-esteem.

3. **Encourage Them To Join A Local Support Group:** Some local and national groups, such as the National Alliance on Mental Illness (NAMI), offer local programs and internet resources that help reduce stigma by educating people who have a mental illness, their families and the general public. Some state and federal agencies, such as those that focus on vocational rehabilitation, and the Department of Veterans Affairs (VA), offer support for people with mental illness.

4. **Get Help At School:** If you or your child has a mental illness that affects learning, find out what plans and programs might help. Discrimination against students because of a mental illness is against the law, and educators at primary, secondary, and college levels are required to accommodate students with mental issues. Talk to teachers, professors or administrators about the best approach and resources. If a teacher doesn't know about a student's disability, it can lead to discrimination, barriers to learning, and poor grades.

5. **Don't Isolate Yourself:** If you have a mental illness, you may be reluctant to tell anyone about it. Your family, friends, clergy, or members of your community can offer you support if

they know about your mental illness. Reach out to people you trust for the compassion, support and the understanding you need.

6. Don't Equate Yourself With Your Illness: You are not the illness. So instead of saying "I'm bipolar," say "I have bipolar disorder." Instead of calling yourself "a schizophrenic," say "I have schizophrenia."

7. Speak Out Against Stigma: Consider expressing your opinions at events, in letters to the editor, or on the internet. It can help instill courage in others facing similar challenges, and educate the public about mental illness.

8. Don't Give Up: Never give up regardless of your situation. The answers to your problems are out there; however, you must find those answers. You will not get better if you sit on the couch, and don't make an effort to get better. You need to know that you will eventually get better. Do not lose hope during the worse of times. Your problems will not last forever, and things do eventually change for the better.

9. Learn To Take It One Day At A Time: Instead of worrying about how you will get through the rest of the week or coming month, try to focus on today. Each day can provide us with different opportunities to learn new things, and that includes learning how to deal with your problems. When the time comes, hopefully you will have learned the skills to deal with your situation.

10. Stand Your Ground: It is important to stand your ground when dealing with family members and coworkers who are giving you a hard time. Explain your situation and your feelings to the people in your life, however don't let them hassle you. Again, your number one priority is to get better, not to please everyone that you surround yourself with.

11. Watch Who You Surround Yourself With: It is important to surround yourself with positive people. Try to keep your distance from those people who are giving you a difficult time. Remember your goal is to remain positive and hopeful. Do not let the negative people in your life bring you down.

12. **Don't Argue With Others:** It is important that you do not get into arguments with those who are giving you a hard time. Your number one priority is to overcome your mental health issues. It is not your job to convince people that you are right and they are wrong. Your health is more important than what other people may think.

13. **Talk To A Counselor:** The most important thing that you need to do is to talk to a counselor about your mental health problems. Seeking professional help will help you to overcome your current issues. In addition, a counselor will be able to give you additional advice on how to deal with your friends and coworkers.

People's judgment of mental patients usually comes form the lack of understanding of the subject. Helping the patient to accept their condition, finding out the best ways to treat the problem, getting support from others, as well as educating others, can go a long way in reducing the stigma faced by individuals with a mental illness.

Chapter 3

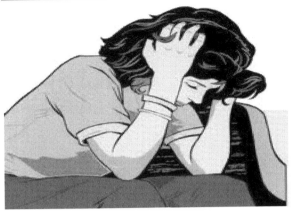

HOW TO STOP MENTAL HEALTH STIGMA

Stigma is one of the most challenging aspects of living with a mental health condition. It causes people to feel ashamed for something that is out of their control, and prevents many from seeking the help they need and speaking out. What is the best way to end mental health stigma?   Here are some of the responses:

Talk openly about mental health. "Mental illness touches so many lives and yet it's STILL a giant secret. Be brave and share your story." --L.L

Educate yourself and others about mental health. "Challenge people respectfully when they are perpetrating stereotypes and misconceptions. Speak up and educate them." –Y.L

Be conscious of your language. "Saying someone is "retarded" or using (or even mentioning) the "N" word is politically incorrect, but it's still fine to throw around words like crazy, psycho, lunatic, etc." –M.C

Encourage e□uality in how people perceive physical illness and mental illness. "We should explain mental illness as similar to any other illness. When someone acts differently or "strange" during diabetic shock we don't blame them for moral failings." –W.N

Show empathy and compassion for those living with a mental health condition. "Love, we can all use more education, but that will not make people change their opinions. When you love and respect people, love and respect all of them. You have a desire to learn more about who they are and what their life is like." –M.W.B

Stop the criminalization of those who live with mental illness. "Professionals and families together need to talk to neighborhood groups, law enforcement, hospitals and legal experts to share experiences and knowledge on interacting with mentally ill." –V.E.J

Push back against the way people who live with mental illness are portrayed in the media: "Push back hard against the media and politicians and pundits that simply deflect real social issues such as gun control to the realm of "psychos" causing mass shootings." –M.C

See the person, not the illness: "Talk about your family and friends with mental illnesses any time a conversation invites the opportunity; with an open heart, love, and real information about the real human being that they are; they are not their condition." –S.S

Advocate for mental health reform. "It's empowering people whenever and wherever you can. It's also writing legislators. It's also talking in front of a board of commissioners to advocate for continued mental health funding... It's doing the right thing and treating others justly." –D.H

Stigma is not something that will go away on its own, but if we work together as a community, we can change the way we perceive mental illness in our society.

Simple Steps to Reduce Stigma about Mental Illness

If you tune into any conversation about mental illness and addiction, it won't be very long until the term "stigma" comes up. Stigma has various definitions, but they all refer to negative attitudes, beliefs, descriptions, language or behavior. In other words, stigma can translate into disrespectful, unfair, or discriminatory patterns in how we think, feel, talk and behave towards individuals experiencing a mental illness.

If you begin to wonder where stigma comes from, that's a complicated question. It's almost like asking where do differences in racial prejudice, political views, religious preference, or sports team allegiances come from. Turns out we are influenced (all too easily) by our family, friends, the media, our culture, environment, inaccurate stereotypes, and a whole host of factors.

Rather than figure out where stigma begins, it's definitely easier to become more aware of what it is and when it occurs. Then we can do our best to educate others about how to reduce stigma, and work towards ultimately eliminating it.

So, how do we become more aware of stigma? It's usually easier to take a look at ourselves first before we try to change the rest of the world. To that end, here's a brief self-assessment quiz on stigma and mental illness. Answer honestly; no one else will need to know your answers.

Mental Illness Stigma Quiz

True or False:

1) There's no real difference between the terms "mentally ill" and "has a mental illness."

2) People with mental illness tend to be dangerous and unpredictable.

3) I would worry about my son or daughter marrying someone with a mental illness.

4) I've made fun of people with mental illness in the past.

5) I don't know if I could trust a co-worker who has a mental illness.

6) I'm scared of, or stay away from people who appear to have a mental illness.

7) People with a mental illness are lazy or weak and need to just "get over it."

8) Once someone has a mental illness, they will never recover.

9) I would hesitate to hire someone with a history of mental illness.

10) I've used terms like "crazy," "psycho," "nut job," or "retarded" in reference to someone with a mental illness.

The scoring is simple; one point for every true response. Unless your score is zero, you have had thoughts, feelings, or behaviors which can contribute to increased stigma toward people with mental illness. The higher your score, the more likely it is you have had these types of experiences. If you scored a zero, congratulate yourself.

How to Reduce Stigma

Now that you've done a □uick self-check and agree there's room for improvement in how we treat people with mental illness, what's next? Well, how about becoming an advocate to reduce mental health stigma right there in your own backyard?

Now you may be saying, "Wait a minute, don't know if I signed on for that." Let's put this into perspective. Have you already signed on to make sure your kids and other passengers in your car wear their seat belts? Did you ever sign on to collect your neighbor's mail while they were on vacation? Have you ever signed on to give a donation to your favorite cause or charity? If so, then you can do this.

But it takes just a little effort. Not too much, just a little. And the rules of the road are ☐uite simple. Here are simple steps you can take as a new mental health stigma fighter:

1) Don't label people who have a mental illness.

Don't say, "He's bipolar" or "she's schizophrenic." People are people, not diagnoses. Instead, say "He has a bipolar disorder" or "She has schizophrenia." And say "has a mental illness" instead of "is mentally ill." All of this is known as "person-first" language, and it's far more respectful, for it recognizes that the illness doesn't define the person.

2) Don't be afraid of people with mental illness.

Sure, they may sometimes display unusual behaviors when their illness is more severe, but people with mental illness aren't more likely to be violent than the general population. In fact, they are more likely to be victims of violence. Don't fall prey to other inaccurate stereotypes, such as the disturbed killer or the weird co-worker depicted in the movies.

3) Don't use disrespectful terms for people with mental illness.

In a research study with British 14-year-olds, the teens came up with over 250 terms to describe mental illness, and the majority were negative. These terms are far too common in our everyday conversations. Also, be careful about using "diagnostic" terms to describe behavior, like "that's my OCD" or "she's so borderline." Given that 1 in 4 adults experience a mental illness, you ☐uite likely may be offending someone and not be aware of it.

4) Don't be insensitive or blame people with mental illness.

It would be silly to tell someone to just "buckle down" and "get over" cancer, and the same applies to mental illness. Also, don't assume that someone is okay just because they look or act okay, or sometimes smile or laugh. Depression, anxiety, and other mental illnesses can often be hidden, but the person can still be in considerable internal distress. Provide support and reassurance when you know someone is having difficulty managing their illness.

5) **Be a role model.**

Stigma is often fueled by lack of awareness and inaccurate information. Model these stigma-reducing strategies through your own comments and behavior, and politely teach them to your friends, family, co-workers, and others in your sphere of influence. Spread the word that treatment works and recovery is possible. Changing attitudes takes time, but repetition is the key, so keep getting the word out to bring about a positive shift in how we treat others.

Former US President Bill Clinton said it very nicely: "Mental illness is nothing to be ashamed of, but stigma and bias shame us all. " Take the next step. Adopt these simple tools, and you can help move the needle in the direction of getting rid of stigma once and for all.

Ways to Cope When a Family Member Has a Mental Illness

Learning that a family member has a mental illness can be both a relief and a shock. Chances are by the time the diagnosis is made, the illness has already created chaos within the family. As in any loss, the first response may be denial, followed by anger, bargaining, depression, and then acceptance. This takes not only a toll on the person with the illness; it affects the entire family.

Unfortunately, there is still a stigma attached to most mental illnesses. Although scientific research has proven otherwise, many people misunderstand and place blame on society or family. Furthermore, finding the right treatment can be a lengthy, expensive process, and the future often seems uncertain. In the midst of stress and anxiety, however, there are several ways for family members to cope, and to make life easier for their loved one, as well.

Any illness takes its toll on a family, but this is even truer with a mental illness. Every member of the family needs support. Whether this consists of a network of family and friends, or a formal support group, sharing with others who understand relieves stress and provides much-needed encouragement. Support groups are also a safe place to ask questions and learn about the illness.

Counseling can help the entire family by assuring them their emotions are normal, diffusing existing conflicts, and finding ways to deal with problems caused by the illness. This may take place individually, as a group, or a combination of both. Finding professionals who are open-minded and well-trained is important, and referrals from trustworthy sources are beneficial.

For the sufferer and the family, a good knowledge of the illness, including its symptoms and its treatments, is critical. Thanks to the internet, there is an abundance of data, and many organizations have relevant publications. Nevertheless, discretion should be used when choosing reliable sources.

Living with uncertainty and stress leads to exhaustion and burnout. Practicing self-care is far from selfish. In fact, it is good for everyone involved. Simple things, such as going for a walk, getting a massage, or meeting friends for coffee, revitalize and strengthen caregivers' ability to cope with feelings of frustration and helplessness. Dealing with a mental illness is an ongoing process, and everyone needs a break now and then.

Regardless of personal beliefs, having some type of spiritual practice not only aids in accepting reality, but it also lessens the need to control the outcome. Yoga, meditation, prayer, and exercise are traditional rituals. Energy medicine, like acupuncture, Qigong, and Reiki, are becoming more popular, and even the medical community has begun to embrace the idea of their efficacy. Attitudes toward mental illnesses are gradually changing, and new treatments are becoming available.

Meanwhile, good medical care, an understanding of the illness, and a strong support system make coping with the challenge easier, and hopes for the future brighter.

Chapter 4

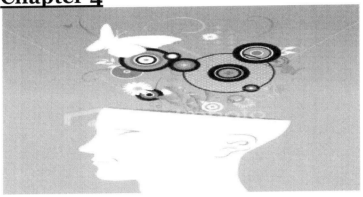

WHAT YOU SHOULD KNOW WHEN DATING SOMEONE WITH A MENTAL ILLNESS

Despite the societal stigma against mental illness, dating someone who has mental illness isn't necessarily all that much different from dating someone who doesn't. They have a wide range of personalities, relationship needs, and baggage, just like people without mental illness. However, here are a few things that are helpful to keep in mind.

This list is designed for individuals who are dating someone who has mental illness, either something they knew about when they started dating, or something that came up after they began dating. While some of this may apply to married relationships or relationships with kids.

1. Communicate with your partner about their illness

Nothing can replace straightforward communication. Let your partner describe their illness in their own words, to whatever extent they're comfortable sharing. Ask them what challenges they commonly experience, and how you can help.

When having this conversation, make sure you're being clear that you're asking to help support them, and that if they aren't comfortable having this conversation right now, that's okay.

You can help make it more of a two-way street by offering some challenges you have, or things you are particularly sensitive about. The goal is to let them share what they're comfortable sharing to help you two have a stronger relationship, not to pick every detail about their mental illness out of them.

2. Educate yourself about their mental illness.

Learning more about your partner's mental illness without putting them in a bad situation can also help you better understand them and their needs. It's not a substitute for talking to them, but it's a good complement.

That said, when reading up on a mental illness, keep in mind that a lot of sources are coming from the perspective of people who don't have mental illness, and as such they sometimes overblow the severity of mental illness or make inaccurate generalizations. Reading can provide a valuable introduction to mental illness, but even the same illness may manifest in different ways in different individuals, so it's not a substitute for your partner's lived experience.

3. Remember they are people first

People with mental illness are people first. They have interests, strengths, and weaknesses, and aren't defined solely by their illness.

Trust your partner first and foremost, both about themselves and about their mental health. Different people with the same mental illness may have different needs, and almost certainly have some different experiences.

If you've been dating for a while, and you recently found out your partner has a mental illness, you might feel uncertain or surprised. If you do, try to remind yourself of what you like about them, and all the strong parts of your relationship. The good things won't change just because your partner has mental illness. In many cases, getting a diagnosis is a good thing, not a bad thing; identifying mental illness can help people manage their illness, and improve their ⬜uality of life.

4. Set Boundaries and Take care of Yourself

Healthy boundaries are important in all relationships, but especially when you're in a romantic relationship. As a society, we have a lot of assumptions about boundaries in relationships, but rarely discuss them. Always advocate for straightforward discussions about boundaries, but it's particularly vital for a healthy relationship when one person (or both) has mental illness.

Even if you're dating someone with mental illness, you need to remember that you aren't your partner's therapist. While expecting some emotional support and comfort in a relationship is reasonable, even healthy, you shouldn't be the sole provider of such support and comfort. You can be there for your partner without letting it take over your life, and if it does start to take over your life, you'll need to have the difficult, but important conversation of setting boundaries.

Not everyone is in a place where they're emotionally ready to be in a healthy relationship (something which applies to both people with and people without mental illness). If someone is being abusive, you do not owe them a relationship, and you should prioritize getting out safely, regardless of whether they have a mental illness or not. Ultimately, you need to take care of yourself. You're in a relationship; you aren't their therapist or caretaker, and you shouldn't have to be.

While mental illness can make relationships tough, everyone comes into a relationship with some sort of baggage. If you communicate well with your partner, and do your part to learn about mental illness, respect your partner, and establish boundaries, mental illness alone doesn't need to be a deal breaker in your relationship.

Chapter 5

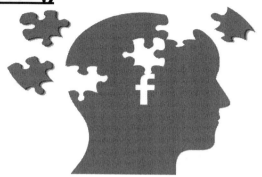

HOW TO DISCLOSE YOUR MENTAL HEALTH PROBLEM

Stress has become an inevitable part of everyone's life these days. With hectic work schedules and daunting deadlines to meet, most people have got accustomed to living pressured lives. In such a fast-paced world, it is not easy for a person to have control over the rapidly changing circumstances, which has an adverse impact on his or her mind and body.

Conse☐uently, in this ever-growing tussle, more and more people are getting exposed to various mental health conditions, such as anxiety and depression, which prevent them from fulfilling their potential. Sadly, not many people get help for their mental issues due to the stigma and myths surrounding such disorders. Moreover, a majority of patients hesitate to discuss and share their mental health concerns with others, which often leads to a delay in seeking medical help.

As a result, many continue to struggle with their condition without any help and support, ultimately leading to chronic disabilities and life-threatening conditions. One can combat the crippling symptoms by following basic self-help techni☐ues. But first of all, one must be upfront to discuss his or her mental issues with a loved one so that ade☐uate steps could be taken to alleviate the risks. Listed below are some tips that can help an individual to open up about his or her mental illness:

Deciding whether to disclose or not: The first thought would certainly be "let's not do it." Talking about one's own mental condition can be tough, considering the negativity prevailing in the society regarding the issue. However, it is important to overcome this denial, and be courageous to speak up about one's mental health condition, and then seek medical help at the earliest.

Selecting a confidante: The society at large lacks knowledge and information concerning mental health. Due to this, most mental disorders are surrounded by myths, misconceptions, marginalization and stigma. Apparently, not everyone understands the plight of a person fighting a serious mental health condition. Therefore, it is important to look for some trustworthy people who can understand the real concerns, while keeping the sufferer's confidentiality intact.

Deciding when to discuss the issue: It is better to confide in someone before the situation goes out of control. While opening up about one's condition with friends or loved ones, it is important to select a person who is most willing to help and provide the needed support. Making oneself comfortable and decluttering the mind before initiating a conversation with a person he or she has confidence in can go a long way in creating a positive environment.

Explaining your struggle: Once someone decides to confront the situation upfront, the next important step is to initiate the conversation regarding the struggle that he or she is dealing with. It is always beneficial to let the person know beforehand about the significance of the discussion so that he or she comes prepared for it.

However, one must keep in mind that throughout the conversation, it is not mandatory for someone to share every details with one's confidante. Instead, one should only share the things he or she is comfortable sharing, and choose to keep intrinsic details private.

Chapter 6

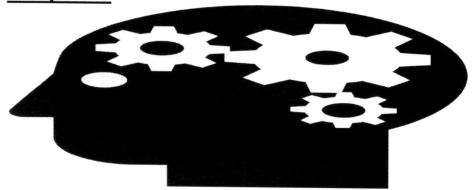

HOW TO TALK TO YOUR TEEN ABOUT MENTAL HEALTH

As children grow and go through a wide range of physical, mental, and emotional changes, it can become more and more difficult to distinguish between normal teenage "moodiness" and a legitimate mental health concern. Teens are often not able to articulate their thoughts and emotions easily, which makes it understandable that teens don't usually express their experiences to their parents. However, a parent could start a conversation that might help protect a teen's well-being and future. For some teens that are really struggling, a conversation with a parent could be absolutely necessary.

The most dominant mental health disorder in adolescence is depression. Although the exact cause of the rise in depression is unknown, contributing factors such as school transitions, social and academic stressors, hormonal changes, family history of mental health disorders, and early traumatic experiences have been identified as major triggers. We must also consider the existential ☐uestions that their developing brain begins to investigate during these challenging times. Such ☐uestions as, "Who am I? Where have I come from? Why am I here?" and, "Where am I going?" add to the intensity of their struggles.

If you believe your teen may be struggling with signs of depression or has a significant change in behavior, the best thing that can be done is to let him/her know that you have noticed some changes, and that you are available to listen to what they are going through. Refrain from asking too many ☐uestions, do not push too hard, and let them know that you will be available when they are ready to talk.

Keep in mind that what you are dealing with might not be logical at first; after all, how anyone would make sense of a teenager's seemingly moody behavior? Therefore, the conversation that you initiate must come from a compassionate, caring, and loving place. Asking, "Why?" typically does not get to the core of the conversation. They probably don't know why they feel the way they do either. Here are a couple of suggestions for an invitation to a dialogue:

"I have noticed you have been ☐uiet lately, I am here any time you want to talk."

"It is okay to be sad, but if you are feeling like this all the time, it's important that I can listen to you share about it."

Validate their feelings and thoughts. It can be very helpful for them to hear acknowledgements, such as "high school can be tough," or "I know you want to be the best you can be," and let them know that it is normal to feel stressed at times.

Generally speaking, teenagers have a short attention span, and might not have patience to talk about such difficult subjects. Time your conversations and know it might take a while for them to share with you. One time that might be ideal to bring up the conversation with them could be while in transit on the way home from school. That time could be comfortable for your teen because they know the conversation will not last long, and they have the control over how much they are ready to share.

Then, once they share, do your best to be content with what they shared, and do not press for more when they are done.

Pushing for more information and conversation could turn them off, and the point is to leave the door open to more conversations.

Most importantly, do not try to talk them out of their mental health issues or explain why they "shouldn't" feel a certain way. Be open and available to listen to their reality. If they share things that are concerning, seek professional help. Start with a conversation with your teen and you might just be a part of helping them work through it.

Chapter 7

HOW TO SUCCEED AT WORK AND MANAGE A MENTAL ILLNESS

We all have that dream for work to be more than just a means to a paycheck, and instead be something that we really love to do. But, if you're someone who suffers from a mental illness or are going through a time that is compromising your mental health (like 1 in 10 people in the world do in their lifetime) you might have a harder time succeeding and achieving your best at work. There are certainly some things you can do to make your work as enjoyable and manageable as possible, no matter what industry you are in.

Choose Your Workplace Wisely

While there might be some elements of your career that are going to be the same no matter where you're working, each company and team will have its own personality, and system for how it functions. Don't decide that one career is not for you just because you don't gel with one particular workplace. You have the potential to be a valuable member of the right team.

Understand Your Environment

When it comes to work, we don't always have a lot of control over our environment, but that doesn't mean that you can't find ways to make your workspace functional for you. If you're someone who needs to be able to have your own ⬜uiet space, find ways to make your office, cubicle, or area as calming as possible. This might mean bringing in some noise-cancelling headphones, or exploring the area around your work where you can take a walk to get away from stress when it does arise.

Don't Keep Your Mental Health a Secret

One of the greatest reasons that a person's mental health can get in the way of their success at work is because they feel that they have to keep their condition a secret from their boss, team, and the company that they work for. But, this might cause you to take more days away from work, and could compromise your ability to do your best when you are present.

There are many workplaces that are now offering a wealth of different resources when it comes to helping their employees cope with mental health issues. But, you can't take advantage of these opportunities if you don't tell the truth. You might find that the company that you work for is not only there to help you through difficult times, but will also make the effort to train others about mental illnesses, helping to reduce the stigma that is still surrounding mental health.

Chapter 8

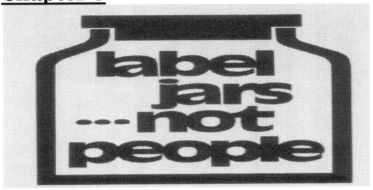

HOW DOES STIGMA AFFECT PEOPLE WITH MENTAL ILLNESS

People with mental health problems experience many different types of stigma. This aspect explores the attitudes and beliefs of the general public towards people with a mental illness, and the lived experiences and feelings of service users and their relatives.

4 key points

- ✓ Stigma can affect many aspects of people's lives.
- ✓ Self-stigma is the process in which people turn stereotypes towards themselves .
- ✓ How the general public perceive people with mental health problems depends on their diagnosis.
- ✓ Stigma can be a barrier to seeking early treatment, cause relapse and hinder recovery.

Stigma can pervade the lives of people with mental health problems in many different ways. It diminishes self-esteem, and robs people of social opportunities. This can include being denied opportunities such as employment or accommodation because of their illness.

Stigma in the form of social distancing has also been observed when people are unwilling to associate with a person with mental illness. This might include not allowing the person to provide childcare, or declining the offer of a date. Self-discrimination or internalized discrimination is the process in which people with mental health problems turn the stereotypes about mental illness adopted by the public, towards themselves. They assume they will be rejected socially, and believe they are not valued.

Being discriminated against has a huge impact on self-esteem and confidence. This can increase isolation from society, and reinforce feelings of exclusion and social withdrawal. Researchers observed that people with mental health problems are "fre□uently the object of ridicule or derision, and are depicted within the media as being violent, impulsive and incompetent". It also found that the myth surrounding violence has not been dispelled, despite evidence to the contrary.

The Media

The media have often been accused of sensationalism by portraying mental illness inaccurately in their □uest to gain higher ratings. However, the media can also play an important role in reaching out to many different audiences to promote mental health literacy. Celebrities such as Stephen Fry (diagnosed with bipolar disorder) have spoken publicly about their illness, and this seems to be effective in reducing stigma.

However, the lived experiences of mental health service users tell a different story to the findings on public attitudes. Service users said they experienced stigmatizing attitudes and behaviors in many aspects of their lives. Common themes emerged across the articles. Many people felt stigmatized as soon as they were diagnosed with a mental illness, and attributed this to the way in which their illness had been portrayed in the media. Receiving a stigmatizing label has such a negative effect on people that the Japanese Society of Psychiatry and Neurology at the demand of the patients' families group changed the name of schizophrenia from "mind-split-disease" to "integration disorder" .

Employment

Many people with mental health problems experienced discrimination when applying for jobs. This included trying to explain gaps in their CV due to episodes of mental ill health. They not only experienced stigma when applying for jobs, but also found that when returning to work colleagues treated them differently, with some experiencing bullying, ridicule, and demotion.

Service users also faced the dilemma of whether to disclose their illness to friends, family, colleagues or future employers. Many felt they could tell their partner or parents about having a mental illness and still feel supported, but only 12% felt able to tell colleagues.

Social Stigma

Individuals who use mental health services reported social discrimination in the community, giving accounts of being physically and verbally attacked by strangers and neighbors, their property being vandalized, or being barred from shops and pubs; those with addictions or psychotic illness tended to experience this more than those with non-psychotic illness. Researches also included examples of being spoken to as if they were stupid or like children, being patronizing, or in some instances, having questions addressed to those accompanying them rather than the individual using the service.

Also, an individual using mental services felt a range of emotions surrounding their experiences of discrimination, including anger, depression, fear, anxiety, isolation, guilt, embarrassment, and above all, hurt.

Health and Relationships

Individuals also encountered discrimination when accessing services such as general partisinors (GPs). Researchers reported professionals as being dismissive or assuming that physical presentations were "all in the mind". This can result in reluctance to return for further visits, which can have a detrimental effect on physical health. This is especially significant, as evidence suggests people with mental illness are at greater risk from physical health problems, including cardiovascular disease, diabetes, obesity and respiratory disease; they also have a higher risk of premature death.

Developing mental illness can also lead to breakdowns in relationships with partners, family and friends. Research reported that a □uarter of children had been teased or bullied because of their parents' mental health problems. Evidence shows rates of drug and alcohol use for self medicating, and psychiatric problems are believed to be rising.

Implications for Nursing

Stigma can affect many aspects of a persons life. Even a brief episode of mental illness can have far-reaching effects on wellbeing, disrupting work, families, relationships and social interactions, impacting on the health and wellbeing not just of patients, but also of their families and friends. This can lead to further psychiatric problems such as anxiety and depression.

Stigma can be a barrier to seeking early treatment; often people will not seek professional help until their symptoms have become serious. Others disengage from services, therapeutic interventions, or stop taking medication, all of which can cause relapse and hinder recovery.

If mental illness is treated early enough, it can reduce further ill health, and ultimately the risk of suicide. By intervening at the earliest possible opportunity, people may be able to avoid a full episode of mental illness, and retain their jobs, relationships or social standing.

It is therefore imperative to reduce the stigma surrounding mental health, and stop these factors impinging on people's mental wellbeing.

Chapter 9

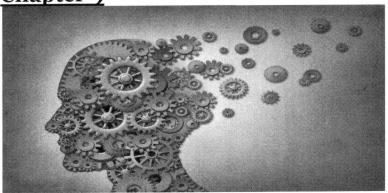

BUILDING AWARENESS AND UNDERSTANDING MENTAL ILLNESS

Mental illness can strike anyone! It knows no age limits, economic status, race, creed, or color. During the course of a year, more than 54 million Americans are affected by one or more mental disorders. Medical science has made incredible progress over the last century in helping us understand, curing and eliminating the causes of many diseases including mental illnesses. However, while doctors continue to solve some of the mysteries of the brain, many of its functions remain a puzzle.

Even at the leading research centers, no one fully understands how the brain works or why it malfunctions. However, researchers have determined that many mental illnesses are probably the result of chemical imbalances in the brain. These imbalances may be inherited, or may develop because of excessive stress or substance abuse.

It is sometimes easy to forget that our brain, like all of our other organs, is vulnerable to disease. People with mental illnesses often exhibit many types of behaviors such as extreme sadness and irritability, and in more severe cases, they may also suffer from hallucinations, and total withdrawal. Instead of receiving compassion and acceptance, people with mental illnesses may experience hostility, discrimination, and stigma.

Why Does Stigma Still Exist?

Unfortunately, the media is responsible for many of the misconceptions which is presented about people with mental illnesses. Newspapers, in particular, often stress a history of mental illness in the backgrounds of people who commit crimes of violence.

Newspapers, in particular, often stress a history of mental illness in the backgrounds of people who commit crimes of violence. Television news programs fre□uently sensationalize crimes where persons with mental illnesses are involved.

Comedians make fun of people with mental illnesses, using their disabilities as a source of humor. Also, national advertisers use stigmatizing images as promotional gimmicks to sell products.

Ironically, the media also offers our best hope for eradicating stigma because of its power to educate and influence public opinion.

What Is A Mental Illness?

A mental illness is a disease that causes mild to severe disturbances in thinking, perception and behavior. If these disturbances significantly impair a person's ability to cope with life's ordinary demands and routines, then he or she should immediately seek proper treatment with a mental health professional. With the proper care and treatment, a person can recover and resume normal activities.

Many mental illnesses are believed to have biological causes, just like cancer, diabetes and heart disease, but some mental disorders are caused by a person's environment and experiences.

THE FIVE MAJOR CATEGORIES OF MENTAL ILLNESS

•Anxiety Disorders

Anxiety disorders are the most common mental illnesses. The three main types are: phobias, panic disorders, and obsessive-compulsive disorders. People who suffer from phobias experience extreme fear or dread from a particular object or situation.

Panic disorders involve sudden, intense feelings of terror for no apparent reason, and symptoms similar to a heart attack. People with obsessive-compulsive disorder try to cope with anxiety by repeating words or phrases or engaging in repetitive, ritualistic behavior such as constant hand washing.

• Mood Disorders

Mood disorders include depression and bipolar disorder (or manic depression) symptoms may include mood swings such as extreme sadness or elation, sleep and eating disturbances, and changes in activity and energy levels. Suicide may be a risk with these disorders.

•Schizophrenia

Schizophrenia is a serious disorder that affects how a person thinks, feels, and acts. Schizophrenia is believed to be caused by chemical imbalances in the brain that produce a variety of symptoms including hallucinations, delusions, withdrawal, incoherent speech and impaired reasoning.

•Dementias

This group of disorders includes diseases like Alzheimer's which leads to loss of mental functions, including memory loss and a decline in intellectual and physical skills.

•Eating Disorders

Anorexia nervosa and bulimia involves serious, potentially life-threatening illnesses. People with these disorders have a preoccupation with food and an irrational fear of being fat. Anorexia is self-starvation while bulimia involves cycles of bingeing (consuming large ⬚uantities of food), and purging (self-inducing vomiting or abusing laxatives). Behavior may also include excessive exercise.

COMMON MISCONCEPTIONS ABOUT MENTAL ILLNESS

Myth: "Young people and children don't suffer from mental health problems."

Fact: It is estimated that more than 6 million young people in America may suffer from a mental health disorder that severely disrupts their ability to function at home, in school, or in their community.

Myth: "People who need psychiatric care should be locked away in institutions."

Fact: Today, most people can lead productive lives within their communities thanks to a variety of supports, programs, and/or medications.

Myth: "A person who has had a mental illness can never be normal."

Fact: People with mental illnesses can recover and resume normal activities. For example, Mike Wallace of "60 Minutes", who has clinical depression, has received treatment and today leads an enriched and accomplished life.

Myth: "Mentally ill persons are dangerous."

Fact: The vast majority of people with mental illnesses are not violent. In the cases when violence does occur, the incidence typically results from the same reasons as with the general public such as feeling threatened or excessive use of alcohol and/or drugs.

Myth: "People with mental illnesses can work low-level jobs, but aren't suited for really important or responsible positions."

Fact: People with mental illnesses, like everyone else, have the potential to work at any level depending on their own abilities, experience and motivation.

HOW TO COMBAT STIGMA

1. Share your experience with mental illness. Your story can convey to others that having a mental illness is nothing to be embarrassed about.

2. Help people with mental illness reenter society. Support their efforts to obtain housing and jobs.

3. Respond to false statements about mental illness or people with mental illnesses. Many people have wrong and damaging ideas on the subject. Accurate facts and information may help change both their ideas and actions.

MENTAL ILLNESS IN THE FAMILY

Recognizing the Warning Signs & How to Cope

Most people believe that mental disorders are rare, and "happen to someone else." Most families are not prepared to cope with learning their loved one has a mental illness. It can be physically and emotionally trying, and can make us feel vulnerable to the opinions and judgments of others.

If you think you or someone you know may have a mental or emotional problem, it is important to remember there is hope and help.

What is mental illness?

A mental illness is a disease that causes mild to severe disturbances in thought and/or behavior, resulting in an inability to cope with life's ordinary demands and routines.

There are more than 200 classified forms of mental illness. Some of the more common disorders are depression, bipolar disorder, dementia, schizophrenia and anxiety disorders. Symptoms may include changes in mood, personality, personal habits and/or social withdrawal.

Mental health problems may be related to excessive stress due to a particular situation or series of events. As with cancer, diabetes and heart disease, mental illnesses are often physical as well as emotional and psychological. Mental illnesses may be caused by a reaction to environmental stresses, genetic factors, biochemical imbalances, or a combination of these. With proper care and treatment many individuals learn to cope or recover from a mental illness, or emotional disorder.

HOW TO COPE DAY-TO-DAY

Accept your feelings

Despite the different symptoms and types of mental illnesses, many families who have a loved one with mental illness, share similar experiences. You may find yourself denying the warning signs, worrying what other people will think because of the stigma, or wondering what caused your loved one to become ill. Accept that these feelings are normal and common among families going through similar situations. Find out all you can about your loved one's illness by reading and talking with mental health professionals. Share what you have learned with others.

Handling unusual behavior

The outward signs of a mental illness are often behavioral. Individuals may be extremely quiet or withdrawn. Conversely, he or she may burst into tears or have outbursts of anger. Even after treatment has started, individuals with a mental illness can exhibit anti-social behaviors.

When in public, these behaviors can be disruptive and difficult to accept.

The next time you and your family member visit your doctor or mental health professional, discuss these behaviors and develop a strategy for coping.

Establishing a support network

Whenever possible, seek support from friends and family members. If you feel you can't discuss your situation with friends or other family members, find a self-help or support group. These groups provide an opportunity for you to talk to other people who are experiencing the same type of problems. They can listen and offer valuable advice.

Seek counseling

Therapy can be beneficial for both the individual with mental illness and other family members. A mental health professional can suggest ways to cope and better understand your loved one's illness.

When looking for a therapist, be patient, and talk to a few professionals so you can choose the person that is right for you and your family. It may take time until you are comfortable, but in the long run you will be glad you took the time.

Taking time out

It is common for the person with the mental illness to become the focus of family life. When this happens, other members of the family may feel ignored or resentful. Some may find it difficult to pursue their own interests.

If you are the caregiver, you need some time for yourself. Schedule time away to prevent becoming frustrated or angry. If you schedule time for yourself it will help you to keep things in perspective, and you may have more patience and compassion for coping or helping your loved one. Only when you are physically and emotionally healthy can you help others.

It is important to remember that there is hope for recovery, and with treatment many people with mental illness return to a productive and fulfilling life.

Warning Signs and Symptoms

To learn more about symptoms that are specific to a particular mental illness, refer to the National Mental Health Association (NMHA) brochure on that illness. The following are signs that your loved one may want to speak to a medical or mental health professional.

In Adults:

Confused thinking

Prolonged depression (sadness or irritability)

Feelings of extreme highs and lows

Excessive fears, worries and anxieties

Social withdrawal

Dramatic changes in eating or sleeping habits

Strong feelings of anger

Delusions or hallucinations

Growing inability to cope with daily problems and activities

Suicidal thoughts

Denial of obvious problems

Numerous unexplained physical ailments

Substance abuse

In Older Children and Pre-Adolescents:

Substance abuse

Inability to cope with problems and daily activities

Change in sleeping and/or eating habits

Excessive complaints of physical ailments

Defiance of authority, truancy, theft, and/or vandalism

Intense fear of weight gain

Prolonged negative mood, often accompanied by poor appetite or thoughts of death

Frequent outbursts of anger

In Younger Children:

Changes in school performance

Poor grades despite strong efforts

Excessive worry or anxiety (i.e. refusing to go to bed or school)

Hyperactivity

Persistent nightmares

Persistent disobedience or aggression

Frequent temper tantrums.

Chapter 10

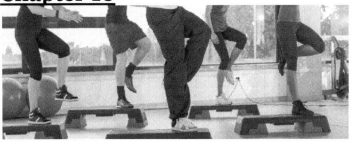

EXERCISE AND MENTAL ILLNESS

Do you remember moping around the house as a kid and mom saying, "Go outside and play"? Mom was onto something. There are numerous studies that indicate exercise is helpful in reducing depression. There is no one identifiable reason as to why it works. So let's look at a few possibilities.

When you exercise, your body releases chemicals called endorphins. Endorphins interact with receptors in your brain and reduce your perception of pain. They also trigger positive feelings in the body. A prime example of the positive feelings that follow a workout would be the "runner's high". Fortunately, it doesn't only occur after running. You can attain that same euphoric feeling through a variety of workouts.

The physical benefits of exercise are as follows:

It lowers blood pressure.

It improves muscle tone and strength.

It strengthens and builds bones.

It strengthens the heart.

It reduces body fat.

It increases energy levels.

It improves the quality of sleep.

While this list is by no means exhaustive, it is clear that our bodies benefit from exercise. Maintaining a healthy body goes a long way, and it could be argued it is vital for a healthy mind.

A note on the improved □uality of sleep - Endorphins also act as sedatives and help with achieving a restful state. Sleep restores the body and mind. There are a multitude of studies that link sleep to healthy brain function.

Another benefit of regular exercise is improved self-esteem. Feeling good about how you look and the way you feel in your body, has a direct impact on self-esteem. The ability to demonstrate self-efficacy through the mastery of exercise improves self-esteem. And like an exercise program, small, attainable victories add up, and the rate of return increases.

One last point that might seem the least important after all of this talk of endorphins, physical benefits, self-esteem, and self-efficacy, but I think might be the key to it all, exercise can be great fun! There are so many different types of exercises. Find the one(s) you like and enjoy. Put all of this together, and of course exercise is helpful in reducing depression.

At home take a holistic, whole body approach to healing that includes balanced meals, 8 hours of sleep nightly, and various opportunities for exercise during the week such as: yoga, dance movement, weight training, swimming, hiking, daily recreation, and group outings.

Conclusion

Thank you again for downloading this book!

As Nietzsche would say, "One must harbor chaos within oneself to give birth to a dancing star," and Aristotle stated, "Why is it that all men who are outstanding in philosophy, poetry, or the arts are so melancholic?"

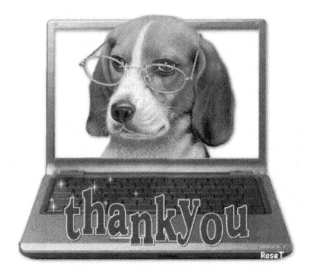

Finally, if you enjoyed this book, then I'd like to ask you for a favor, would you be kind enough to leave a review for this book on Amazon? It'd be greatly appreciated!

Thank you and good luck!

Preview Of 'MENTAL HEALTH STIGMA: HOW TO OVERCOME MENTAL HEALTH STIGMA IN AMERICA'

Chapter 1

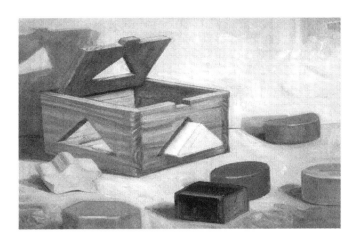

DISCRIMINATION IMPACT OF STIGMAS

Stigma can prompt discrimination. Discrimination may be obvious and immediate, for example, someone making a negative comment about your mental illness or your treatment. On the other hand, it might be unexpected or modest, for example, by keeping away from you because they expect you to be unsteady, savage, or dangerous because of your mental health condition. You may start to judge yourself.

The destructive impact of stigma can include:

- Reluctance to look for help or treatment.

- Stop seeing family, friends, colleagues, or others you know.

- Fewer doors open for employment, school, and social settings.

- Bullying, physical roughness, or aggravation from others.

- Health insurance that doesn't cover your mental health treatment.

- The conviction that you'll never have the capacity to succeed at a specific tasks, or that you can't improve your circumstances.

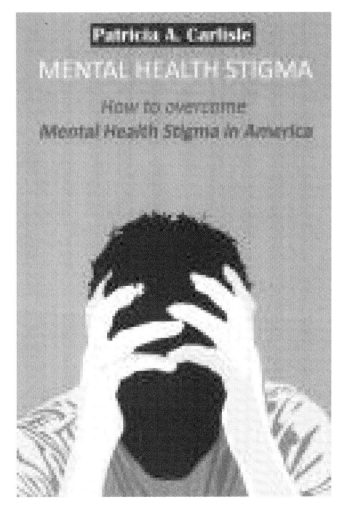

To check out the rest of (MENTAL HEALTH STIGMA: HOW TO OVERCOME MENTAL HEALTH STIGMA IN AMERICA) go to Amazon.com

Check Out My Other Books

Below you'll find some of my other popular books that are popular on Amazon and Kindle as well. Alternatively, you can visit my author page on Amazon to see other work done by me.

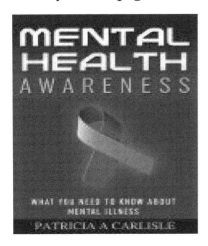

MENTAL HEALTH AWARENESS: WHAT YOU NEED TO KNOW ABOUT MENTAL ILLNESS.

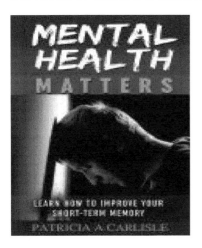

MENTAL HEALTH MATTERS: LEARN HOW TO IMPROVE YOUR SHORT-TERM MEMORY.

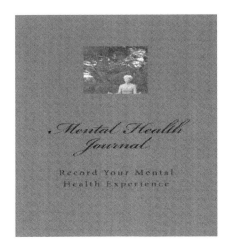

MENTAL HEALTH JOURNAL: RECORD YOUR MENTAL HEALTH EXPERIENCE.

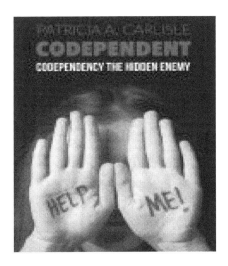

CODEPENDENT: CODEPENDENCY THE HIDDEN ENEMY.

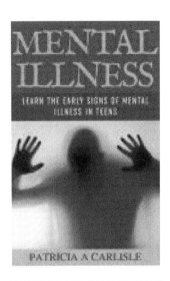

MENTAL ILLNESS: LEARN THE EARLY SIGNS OF MENTAL ILLNESS IN TEENS.

BONUS: SUBSCRIBE TO THE FREE BOOK

Beginners Guide to Yoga & Meditation

"Stressed out? Do You Feel Like The World Is Crashing Down Around You? Want To Take A Vacation That Will Relax Your Mind, Body And Spirit? Well this Easy To Read Step By Step

E-Book Makes It All Possible!"

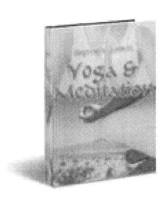

Instructions on how to join our mailing list, and receive a free copy of "Yoga and Meditation" can be found in any of my Kindle eBooks.

NOTES

NOTES

NOTES

NOTES

NOTES

NOTES

Printed in Great Britain
by Amazon